Exploring the Potential of Aromatherapy for Enhancing Cognitive Function and Mental Clarity.

Frank P. Marson

Table of Contents

CHAPTER ONE..4

Introduction 4

Definition of Aromatherapy..................................4

History of Aromatherapy................................6

Benefits of Aromatherapy 9

CHAPTER TWO 12

Essential Oils..12

Types of Essential Oils.................................12

Properties of Essential Oils 15

How to Select Essential Oils............................17

CHAPTER THREE...21

Aromatherapy Techniques 21

Inhalation..21

Topical Application......................................23

Aromatherapy Massage 25

CHAPTER FOUR..29

Safety and Precautions 29

Skin Irritation.................................29

Possible Health Risks.................32

Contraindications 35

CHAPTER FIVE 39

Conclusion...............................39

Summary of Aromatherapy Benefits...............39

Resources and Further Reading.......................41

Final Thoughts 45

CHAPTER ONE

Introduction

Definition of Aromatherapy

Aromatherapy is a holistic healing treatment that uses natural plant extracts to promote health and well-being. The essential oils extracted from flowers, bark, stems, leaves, roots, and other parts of plants are used to enhance psychological and physical well-being. Aromatherapy has been used for centuries in many cultures around the world and is becoming increasingly popular in the modern world.

The practice of aromatherapy is based on the belief that the aroma of essential oils can affect the body, mind, and spirit. Essential oils contain natural compounds that have an effect on the nervous system, hormones, and other organs. Inhaling these compounds through the nose or skin can help to balance the body's natural systems and promote healing.

Aromatherapy is a holistic healing practice that is based on the idea that essential oils can have a beneficial effect on both physical and mental health. The essential oils used in aromatherapy are believed to be able to stimulate certain parts of the brain, which can help to reduce stress, anxiety, and depression. Essential oils can also boost the immune system and improve circulation.

Essential oils are extracted from plants and used in aromatherapy treatments. These oils contain many different compounds, including terpenes, alcohols, aldehydes, and ketones. These compounds are absorbed through the skin and can travel through the bloodstream to the organs. When essential oils are used in aromatherapy, they can be applied topically, inhaled, or diffused in the air. When inhaled, the oils are absorbed through the olfactory system and can affect the brain, hormones, and other organs. Topical application of essential oils can help to relieve pain, reduce inflammation, and stimulate circulation. Aromatherapy is a safe and natural way to promote health and well-being. It can be used to treat a variety of health conditions, including stress, anxiety, depression, and insomnia. It can also be used to improve physical health, including circulation and immune system functioning.

Aromatherapy is a holistic healing practice that is based on the belief that essential oils can have a beneficial effect on both physical and mental health. Essential oils are extracted from plants and used in aromatherapy treatments. These oils contain many different compounds, which are believed to be able to stimulate certain parts of the brain and improve circulation. Aromatherapy can be used to treat a variety of health conditions, including stress, anxiety, depression, and insomnia. It is a safe and natural way to promote health and well-being.

History of Aromatherapy

Aromatherapy is the practice of using fragrant essential oils extracted from plants to promote physical and psychological wellbeing. The use of natural fragrance has been around for centuries, dating back to Ancient Egypt, where essential oils were used for various medicinal, spiritual and cosmetics purposes.

In the early 20th century, French chemist Rene Maurice Gattefosse was the first to use the term 'aromatherapie', having discovered that lavender oil could help heal a burn on his hand. After this, he began experiments to determine the effects of various essential oils on the body.

Gattefosse's work was further developed by French doctor Jean Valnet, who published 'The Practice of Aromatherapy' in 1964. In this book, Valnet detailed the use of essential oils for healing purposes, including the treatment of skin diseases, respiratory problems and digestive complaints.

In the late 1970s, aromatherapy became popular in the West, largely due to the efforts of British aroma therapist and nurse, Marguerite Maury. Maury advocated using essential oils in massage, and developed a system of application. This system is still used today, and involves diluting the essential oil in a carrier oil before applying it to the skin. Since then, aromatherapy has continued to evolve and become increasingly popular. Many people now use essential oils for a variety of purposes, including relaxation, stress relief and pain management. Aromatherapy continues to be researched and developed, with new uses for essential oils being discovered all the time. Today, it is used in a variety of settings, including hospitals, spas, beauty salons and even homes.

Aromatherapy is an incredibly versatile practice that has been used for centuries to promote physical and psychological wellbeing. From ancient Egypt to modern day, essential oils have been used to treat a range of ailments and conditions, and to promote relaxation and stress relief. Thanks to the efforts of pioneers like Rene Maurice Gattefosse and Jean Valnet, aromatherapy continues to be researched and developed, with new uses being discovered all the time.

Benefits of Aromatherapy

Aromatherapy is an alternative medicine practice that utilizes essential oils for healing and stress relief. Essential oils are derived from plants and are used to create a calming and therapeutic atmosphere. Aromatherapy is used to treat a variety of physical and emotional ailments, from headaches to depression. It is believed that the essential oils can be inhaled or applied topically to the skin to create a sense of balance and well-being.

The benefits of aromatherapy are far-reaching and can be applied to a variety of different health conditions. Aromatherapy can help to reduce stress, anxiety, and depression, as well as improve sleep quality and reduce fatigue. The essential oils used can also help to reduce headaches, boost energy levels, and improve concentration. One of the most common benefits of aromatherapy is its ability to reduce stress and anxiety. Aromatherapy can help to create a calming and soothing atmosphere, which can help to reduce feelings of anxiety and stress. The scent of the essential oils can also help to relax the body and mind, allowing the person to relax and let go of any pent-up tension.

Aromatherapy can also help to improve sleep quality. Essential oils such as lavender and chamomile can help to reduce insomnia and promote deeper, more restful sleep. This can help to reduce fatigue and improve energy levels throughout the day. Aromatherapy can also be used to treat physical ailments such as headaches, muscle tension, and even menstrual cramps. Essential oils such as lavender and peppermint can be used to reduce headaches and muscle tension, while chamomile and rose can be used to reduce cramping

Finally, aromatherapy can be used to improve mood and mental clarity. The scents of the essential oils can help to improve focus and concentration, while also lifting mood and promoting a sense of well-being. Essential oils such as lemon and orange can be used to improve alertness and concentration, while lavender and ylang-ylang can be used to reduce feelings of sadness and anxiety.

In conclusion, aromatherapy is a safe and natural way to treat a variety of physical and emotional ailments. The essential oils used in aromatherapy can help to reduce stress, improve sleep quality, reduce headaches, boost energy levels, and improve mood and mental clarity. Aromatherapy is a great option for those looking for an alternative or complementary treatment to traditional medicine.

CHAPTER TWO

Essential Oils

Types of Essential Oils

Essential oils are extracted from plant material, typically from flowers, leaves, roots, and other parts of the plant. They have been used for centuries for medicinal, cosmetic, and spiritual purposes. Essential oils are highly concentrated and are very powerful, so they must be used with care.

There are many different types of essential oils, and each has its own unique properties and uses. Some of the most popular types of essential oils include:

Lavender: Lavender is one of the most popular essential oils, known for its calming and soothing properties. It is often used to reduce stress, anxiety, and insomnia. Lavender can also be used on the skin to help heal cuts, scrapes, and other minor skin irritations.

Peppermint: Peppermint essential oil is known for its cooling, refreshing scent. It is often used to help clear the mind and reduce fatigue. Peppermint can also be used to help relieve muscle pain and headaches.

Eucalyptus: Eucalyptus essential oil has a strong, medicinal scent. It is often used to help clear the lungs and relieve stuffy noses. Eucalyptus can also help to reduce inflammation and reduce joint and muscle pain.

Tea Tree: Tea tree essential oil is known for its antibacterial and antifungal properties. It is often used to help clear acne and other skin conditions. Tea tree can also be used to help treat colds, coughs, and other respiratory infections.

Lemon: Lemon essential oil is known for its fresh, citrus scent. It is often used to help reduce stress and fatigue, as well as to help boost mood. Lemon can also be used to help reduce inflammation and to help treat skin conditions.

Rose: Rose essential oil is known for its sweet, romantic scent. It is often used to help reduce anxiety and promote feelings of love and joy. Rose can also be used to reduce inflammation and to help treat skin conditions.

Bergamot: Bergamot essential oil is known for its citrusy, invigorating scent. It is often used to help reduce stress, depression, and anxiety. Bergamot can also be used to help reduce inflammation and to help treat skin conditions.

Cedarwood: Cedarwood essential oil is known for its woodsy, calming scent. It is often used to help reduce stress, anxiety, and insomnia. Cedarwood can also be used to help reduce inflammation and to help treat skin conditions.

These are just a few of the many types of essential oils available. Each type of oil has its own unique properties and uses, so it is important to research each one before using it. It is also important to use essential oils safely and follow the manufacturer's instructions. Essential oils should never be ingested, and they should always be diluted before being applied to the skin.

Properties of Essential Oils

Essential oils are natural, aromatic compounds extracted from plants and herbs. They have been used for centuries to treat medical conditions, to promote relaxation, and for healing and spiritual purposes. Essential oils are also gaining popularity for their many health benefits, including their ability to reduce stress and anxiety, improve mood, and support immune and digestive health. Essential oils are made up of small molecules and are easily absorbed by the skin. This makes them very effective in aromatherapy, massage, and natural skin care. Essential oils are also used in a variety of other ways, such as in cleaning products, as insect repellents, and as a natural fragrance.

Essential oils have various properties that make them beneficial for therapeutic use. One of the most important properties is their ability to penetrate the skin easily. This allows the essential oil to reach the bloodstream quickly, where it can be used to treat a variety of medical conditions.

The second important property of essential oils is their high concentration of volatile compounds. Volatile compounds are the active ingredients in essential oils, and they are responsible for the therapeutic benefits of the oils. By releasing these compounds into the air, essential oils are able to work their magic quickly and effectively. Essential oils are also known for their antimicrobial properties. When applied to the skin, essential oils can help to kill bacteria, fungi, and viruses. This makes them useful for treating skin infections, as well as for preventing the spread of infection. Essential oils are also used for their soothing and calming effects. When inhaled, certain essential oils can help to reduce stress and promote relaxation. This can be helpful for people who are dealing with anxiety, depression, or insomnia.

Finally, essential oils are known for their ability to boost the immune system. By fighting free radicals and providing antioxidants, essential oils can help to protect the body against infection and disease.

In conclusion, essential oils are a powerful and versatile tool that can be used for a variety of purposes. From treating medical conditions to promoting relaxation and boosting immunity, essential oils are a natural and effective way to improve your health and wellbeing.

How to Select Essential Oils

Essential oils have been used for centuries for their therapeutic properties, and today, they are becoming increasingly popular as a natural alternative to modern medicine. Selecting the right essential oil can be an overwhelming task, but with a bit of knowledge and guidance, you can make an informed and effective choice.

When selecting an essential oil, it is important to consider its therapeutic benefits. Every oil has unique properties and can be used to treat a variety of health issues. For instance, lavender oil is often used to treat depression and anxiety, while peppermint oil can relieve nausea and headaches. It's important to select the oil that best suits your needs.

It is also essential to consider the source of the oil. When selecting an oil, make sure it is from a reputable source. Look for organic, wild-crafted, and steam-distilled essential oils. These oils are free of chemicals and synthetics, making them safer for use. It's also important to select oils that are free of any additives, such as carrier oils and fragrances. In addition, it's important to select essential oils that are of a high quality. To ensure quality, you should look for oils that are certified pure therapeutic grade. This certification guarantees that the oil is of a high quality and is suitable for use in aromatherapy. When selecting essential oils, it's important to take into account their therapeutic properties. Different oils have different properties, so it's important to select the right oil for your specific needs. For example, lavender and chamomile are both calming and relaxing, while eucalyptus and rosemary are both energizing. Once you have selected an essential oil, it's important to dilute it properly. Essential oils are highly concentrated and should not be used directly on the skin. Instead, they should be mixed with a carrier oil, such as almond or coconut oil, to reduce their strength and make them more suitable for topical use.

Finally, it is important to consider the cost of essential oils. Essential oils can range in price from very inexpensive to quite expensive, depending on the brand, source, and quality. In general, it's best to select an essential oil that is within your budget and meets your needs.

Selecting essential oils can be a daunting task, but with a bit of research and guidance, you can make an informed and effective choice. Before selecting an oil, research its therapeutic benefits, source, and quality. Make sure to purchase oils that are certified pure therapeutic grade and to dilute them properly with a suitable carrier oil. Finally, consider the cost of the oil and select one that is within your budget. With these tips, you can confidently select an essential oil that will be beneficial to your health and wellbeing.

CHAPTER THREE

Aromatherapy Techniques

Inhalation

Inhalation is a form of aromatherapy that involves the use of essential oils and other aromatic substances for their therapeutic effects. The aromas of these substances are inhaled directly or through the use of a diffuser, which disperses the essential oils into the air. Inhalation is one of the most popular and effective forms of aromatherapy, as it allows the user to directly experience the therapeutic benefits of the essential oils.

When essential oils are inhaled, they stimulate certain receptors in the nose and brain, known as olfactory receptors. These receptors then send signals to the brain, which can then affect mood, emotions, and other physiological effects. Depending on the essential oil that is inhaled, the effects can range from calming and soothing to energizing and invigorating.

Inhalation can be done in several ways. One of the simplest and most common methods is to simply smell the essential oils directly from the bottle. This can be done with a few drops of the essential oil placed onto a cloth or cotton ball, or by using a diffuser such as an aromatherapy lamp or candle burner. Inhalation can also be done through the use of a steam inhaler, which disperses the essential oils into the air via steam. Inhalation is a great way to experience the therapeutic benefits of essential oils. However, it is important to remember that essential oils are highly concentrated and should be used with caution. Inhaling essential oils can cause irritation to the respiratory tract and should be avoided if you have a respiratory condition such as asthma. It is also important to be aware of the potential side effects of certain essential oils, as some may cause an allergic reaction.

Inhalation is a powerful tool for aromatherapy, and is a great way to experience the therapeutic benefits of essential oils. When used properly, inhalation can help to reduce stress and anxiety, improve sleep, and promote relaxation. Inhalation is also a great way to experience the aromas of different essential oils, allowing users to find the ones that they enjoy the most. By combining inhalation with other forms of aromatherapy, such as massage or topical application, the therapeutic benefits of essential oils can be maximized.

Topical Application

Aromatherapy is an ancient healing practice that uses essential oils to promote health and wellbeing. Topical application is one of the most popular methods of administering essential oils, as it is a safe and effective way to deliver the therapeutic benefits of the oils to the body.

Topical application involves applying essential oils directly to the skin. This can be done with a massage oil, lotion, or other carrier oil like sweet almond oil. The essential oils are usually diluted before being applied, as they can be powerful and can cause irritation if used neat (undiluted).

When using essential oils topically, it is important to take into consideration the individual's skin type. Those with sensitive skin should use a carrier oil to dilute the oil, and be sure to use only a few drops of the essential oil. It is also important to avoid using essential oils on broken or irritated skin. Topical application of essential oils can be used to reduce stress, lift mood, and promote relaxation. Lavender is one of the most commonly used essential oils for this purpose, as it has a calming effect on the body and mind. Other oils such as rose, chamomile, and ylang ylang are also known to be effective in reducing stress and promoting relaxation.

Essential oils can also be used to help relieve pain and reduce inflammation. Peppermint oil and eucalyptus oil are two of the most popular oils used for this purpose. When applied topically, they can help to reduce muscle tension and pain, as well as reduce inflammation.

In addition to its therapeutic benefits, topical application of essential oils can also be used to improve skin health. Essential oils such as lavender, rose, and tea tree oil all have antiseptic, antibacterial, and antifungal properties. When applied topically, these oils can help to protect the skin from bacteria, viruses, and fungi. They can also help to reduce skin inflammation, redness, and irritation.

Topical application of essential oils is a simple and effective way to deliver the therapeutic benefits of the oils to the body. It is important to remember to always dilute essential oils before applying them to the skin, and to always consider individual skin types when using essential oils topically. With proper use, topical application of essential oils can help to reduce stress, relieve pain and inflammation, and improve skin health.

Aromatherapy Massage

Aromatherapy massage is a type of massage therapy that incorporates essential oils and plant extracts in order to improve the physical and emotional well-being of the client. Aromatherapy massage is a holistic form of therapy that works to improve the overall health of the individual, while providing a calming and relaxing experience.

Aromatherapy massage has been used for centuries as a natural form of healing. The essential oils used in aromatherapy massage are extracted from plants and herbs, and each scent is believed to have a different therapeutic effect on the body. In aromatherapy massage, the therapist will typically use a combination of essential oils that are selected to address the specific needs of the client. The most common essential oils used in aromatherapy massage are lavender, sandalwood, rose and chamomile. Lavender is known for its calming and soothing effects, while sandalwood helps to reduce stress and anxiety, and rose helps to heal skin irritations. Chamomile, on the other hand, is a natural anti-inflammatory and can help to reduce swelling and discomfort.

When performing an aromatherapy massage, the therapist will begin by applying a blend of essential oils to the client's skin. The essential oils will be gently massaged into the skin using long, flowing strokes, which promotes relaxation and increases circulation. After the oil has been absorbed into the skin, the therapist will then use a variety of massage techniques, such as Swedish massage, deep tissue massage, and Shiatsu, to provide the individual with a deeply therapeutic massage. The benefits of aromatherapy massage are numerous. It can help to reduce stress, relieve muscle tension, improve circulation, and promote relaxation. In addition, aromatherapy massage is believed to boost the immune system, improve mental clarity, and even help with insomnia.

Aromatherapy massage can be used to treat a variety of conditions, including back pain, headaches, menstrual cramps, and digestive disorders. It can also be used to treat emotional issues, such as depression and anxiety

In general, aromatherapy massage is a safe and effective form of therapy for individuals of all ages and health conditions. However, it is important to note that some essential oils can be irritating to sensitive skin, and should be used with caution. Additionally, pregnant women and people with certain medical conditions should consult with a doctor prior to using aromatherapy massage.

Aromatherapy massage is a powerful and relaxing form of therapy that can be used to both improve physical and emotional health. With its calming and healing effects, it can be an invaluable tool for anyone looking to improve their overall well-being.

CHAPTER FOUR

Safety and Precautions

Skin Irritation

Aromatherapy is an ancient practice that uses essential oils extracted from flowers, herbs, fruits, and other plants to improve physical and mental wellbeing. Though this practice has been around for centuries, it is becoming increasingly popular in modern times as people look for natural solutions to their health problems. While essential oils can provide many benefits, they can also cause skin irritation if they are not used correctly.

Skin irritation is a common side effect of aromatherapy, and it can range from mild to severe. Mild irritation can cause redness, itching, and burning sensations on the skin. In more serious cases, it can lead to rashes, blistering, and hives. There are several causes of skin irritation from aromatherapy, including:

• Sensitivity to an essential oil or other ingredient used in the blend.

• Allergic reactions to an essential oil or other ingredient.

• Improper dilution of the essential oil in a carrier oil, such as coconut or almond oil.

• Applying the essential oil directly to the skin without properly diluting it.

• Using essential oils that are not suitable for topical use.

• Using essential oils in combination with certain medications or other skin care products. In order to reduce the risk of skin irritation, it is important to properly dilute essential oils in a carrier oil before applying them to the skin. It is also important to use only essential oils that are suitable for topical use, as not all essential oils are safe to be applied directly to the skin. If you are using a combination of essential oils, it is important to make sure that the oils are compatible and that they will not cause any skin irritation when used together. It is also important to be aware of any allergies or sensitivities that you may have to an essential oil or other ingredient used in the blend. If you are sensitive to an essential oil, it is best to avoid using it altogether or to use an alternative oil in its place. When using essential oils on the skin, it is important to pay attention to any changes in your skin, such as redness, itching, or burning. If you experience any of these symptoms, you should immediately remove the essential oil and wash the area with warm water and soap. If the irritation persists, it is best to seek medical advice.

In summary, skin irritation is a common side effect of aromatherapy. It can range from mild to severe and can be caused by a variety of factors, such as sensitivity to an essential oil or other ingredient, improper dilution of the essential oil, or using an essential oil that is not suitable for topical use. To reduce the risk of skin irritation, it is important to properly dilute essential oils in a carrier oil before applying them to the skin and to use only essential oils that are suitable for topical use. If you experience any skin irritation from using essential oils, it is best to remove the oil and seek medical advice if necessary.

Possible Health Risks

Aromatherapy is a type of alternative medicine that uses essential oils and other aromatic plant compounds with the aim of improving physical and mental health. It is believed to work by stimulating the olfactory system, which affects the limbic system of the brain and can influence the body's hormones and other physiological functions.

Aromatherapy is generally considered safe and is often used to treat a variety of ailments, including anxiety and depression, insomnia, skin conditions, muscle pain, and headaches. However, when used improperly or without the guidance of a qualified aroma therapist, it can lead to a number of serious health risks.

The first potential risk of aromatherapy is allergic reactions. Essential oils, which are highly concentrated, can cause skin irritation and allergic reactions. These reactions can range from mild to severe, and can even be life-threatening in some cases. Therefore, it is important to be aware of the potential for allergic reactions when using aromatherapy, and to take the necessary precautions, such as patch testing, to avoid them.

Another potential risk of aromatherapy is skin sensitivity. Essential oils can be very potent and can cause skin sensitivity if used in concentrations that are too high. This is especially true for individuals with sensitive skin, such as those with eczema. Therefore, it is important to be aware of the potential for skin sensitivity and to use the oils in their recommended dilutions. In addition, aromatherapy can cause adverse reactions if used incorrectly or without the guidance of a qualified aromatherapist. For instance, some essential oils should not be used during pregnancy, and some can be toxic if ingested. Therefore, it is important to be aware of the potential risks and to consult a qualified aromatherapist before using any essential oils.

Finally, it is important to note that some essential oils should not be used undiluted. Undiluted essential oils can cause skin irritation, allergic reactions, and even chemical burns. Therefore, it is important to always use essential oils in the recommended dilutions.

In conclusion, aromatherapy is generally considered safe and can be beneficial for a variety of ailments. However, it is important to be aware of the potential health risks associated with it, such as allergic reactions, skin sensitivity, and adverse reactions if used incorrectly or without the guidance of a qualified aromatherapist. Therefore, it is important to take the necessary precautions and to always consult a qualified aromatherapist before using essential oils.

Contraindications

Aromatherapy is a holistic healing treatment that uses natural plant extracts to promote health and well-being. Essential oils, the main component of aromatherapy, are highly concentrated, volatile liquids that are extracted from aromatic plants and herbs. They are used for a variety of therapeutic purposes, including relaxation, stress relief, pain relief, and mood enhancement.

However, aromatherapy is not recommended for everyone and there are certain precautions to be taken. One of the most important considerations is the contraindications of aromatherapy. A contraindication is a situation in which a particular treatment or procedure should not be used because it may be harmful to the patient.

Contraindications in aromatherapy can be divided into two categories: physical and psychological. Physical contraindications are those related to an individual's health and physiology, while psychological contraindications are related to an individual's mental or emotional state.

Physical contraindications in aromatherapy include pregnancy, epilepsy, cancer, heart disease, high blood pressure, asthma, diabetes, and a weakened immune system. Aromatherapy should not be used on pregnant women because of the potential for essential oils to be absorbed into the skin and travel through the placenta. Additionally, essential oils can increase the risk of seizures for those with epilepsy, and can irritate the respiratory system for those with asthma. Those with weakened immune systems should avoid aromatherapy as the essential oils can further weaken the immune system. It is also important to check with a physician prior to using aromatherapy if you have any of the above conditions.

Psychological contraindications in aromatherapy include mental health disorders such as depression, anxiety, bipolar disorder, and schizophrenia. Essential oils can be used to treat symptoms of these conditions, but they can also trigger episodes of mania or psychosis. Additionally, those who have recently experienced a traumatic event should avoid aromatherapy, as the powerful scents can be too overwhelming. It is important to be honest with your aroma therapist about your psychological state prior to using aromatherapy.

In addition to physical and psychological contraindications, there are also certain allergic reactions that can occur as a result of using essential oils. Those with sensitive skin, allergies, or a history of allergies should avoid certain essential oils, as they may cause skin irritation or an allergic reaction. It is important to speak to your aroma therapist about any allergies or sensitivities prior to using essential oils.

In conclusion, aromatherapy is a safe and effective treatment when used correctly and with the proper precautions. While it is generally safe, there are certain contraindications that should be considered. Those who are pregnant, have epilepsy, cancer, heart disease, high blood pressure, asthma, diabetes, or a weakened immune system should not use aromatherapy. Additionally, those with mental health disorders and those who have recently experienced a traumatic event should avoid aromatherapy. Lastly, those with allergies or sensitivities should speak to their aroma therapist about any potential allergic reactions. By following these guidelines, aromatherapy can be a safe and effective treatment for promoting health and well-being.

CHAPTER FIVE

Conclusion

Summary of Aromatherapy Benefits

Aromatherapy is an ancient practice of using essential oils to improve physical and psychological health. It has been used for centuries in many cultures, and is becoming increasingly popular today. Aromatherapy is the therapeutic use of essential oils and plant extracts to promote physical and psychological well-being. Essential oils are derived from plants, flowers, roots, and leaves, and are highly concentrated, aromatic compounds that have been used for centuries as a means of healing and promoting health.

Aromatherapy is believed to work by stimulating the olfactory system, which is responsible for our sense of smell. The aroma of essential oils can evoke a wide range of emotions, such as relaxation, alertness, and calm. When essential oils are inhaled, they enter the bloodstream and travel throughout the body, providing a variety of healing benefits.

The primary benefits of aromatherapy are that it helps to reduce stress and anxiety, improve sleep, reduce inflammation, and alleviate pain. Aromatherapy has been studied and found to be effective in reducing stress and anxiety, and promoting relaxation. Studies have shown that aromatherapy can reduce the physical and emotional symptoms of stress and anxiety, including headaches, insomnia, and restlessness. It can also be used to help improve mood and reduce feelings of depression and fatigue. In addition to its stress-relieving effects, aromatherapy can also be used to reduce inflammation, which can help alleviate pain. Essential oils have anti-inflammatory properties that can reduce swelling and pain caused by arthritis, muscle strain, and other conditions.

Aromatherapy can also be used to enhance sleep. Essential oils such as lavender and chamomile are believed to help relax the body and mind, making it easier to fall asleep. Aromatherapy can also be used to boost energy levels and improve concentration, allowing people to stay alert and productive throughout the day.

Overall, aromatherapy is a safe and effective way to improve physical and psychological health. Essential oils are highly concentrated, so it is important to dilute them in a carrier oil before applying them to the skin. Aromatherapy should not be used in place of conventional medicine, but it can be used as an adjunct therapy to promote relaxation and well-being.

Resources and Further Reading

Aromatherapy is a form of alternative medicine which uses essential oils to improve physical and mental well-being. It is believed that these essential oils have healing properties which can help to relax the mind and body, reduce stress, improve mood, and even treat certain medical conditions. Aromatherapy is often used in combination with other forms of alternative medicine such as massage, reflexology, and acupuncture.

When it comes to aromatherapy, there are many resources and further readings available to those looking to learn more about the practice. Here are some of the best resources and further readings for aromatherapy:

1. Aromatherapy Books: There are many books available on the subject of aromatherapy. These books provide readers with an in-depth look at the history, science, and uses of essential oils. Some of the more popular books include "The Complete Guide to Aromatherapy" by Valerie Ann Worwood and "Aromatherapy for Health Professionals" by Sharon Falsetto.

2. Aromatherapy Websites: There are many websites available which provide information on aromatherapy. These websites often provide information on different types of essential oils, their uses, and safety tips. Some of the more popular websites include Aromaweb.com, Aroma-Zone.com, and Aromatics International.

3. Aromatherapy Magazines: There are many magazines dedicated to aromatherapy. These magazines often provide information on different essential oils, their uses, and safety tips. Some of the more popular magazines include Aromatherapy Today, Aromatherapy Times, and The Essential Oil Magazine.

4. Aromatherapy Blogs: There are many blogs dedicated to aromatherapy. These blogs often provide information on different essential oils, their uses, and safety tips. Some of the more popular blogs include Aromatherapy for All and Aromatherapy World.

5. Aromatherapy Videos: There are many videos available on the subject of aromatherapy. These videos often provide information on different essential oils, their uses, and safety tips. Some of the more popular videos include Aromatherapy for Beginners, Aromatherapy for Relaxation, and Aromatherapy for Stress Relief.

6. Aromatherapy Conferences and Seminars: There are many conferences and seminars dedicated to aromatherapy. These conferences and seminars often provide information on different essential oils, their uses, and safety tips. Some of the more popular conferences and seminars include the International Aromatherapy Conference, the National Association for Holistic Aromatherapy Conference, and the World Aromatherapy Congress.

7. Aromatherapy Schools and Courses: There are many schools and courses dedicated to aromatherapy. These schools and courses often provide information on different essential oils, their uses, and safety tips. Some of the more popular schools and courses include Aromatherapy Associates, Aromahead Institute, and Pacific Institute of Aromatherapy.

These are just a few of the many resources and further readings available for those looking to learn more about aromatherapy. By taking advantage of these resources, readers can gain a better understanding of the practice and learn how to safely and effectively use essential oils for their own personal health and wellness.

Final Thoughts

Aromatherapy is a natural form of healing that dates back centuries and has been used to treat a variety of ailments from physical to emotional. It is a form of alternative medicine that uses essential oils to promote healing, relaxation and balance. Essential oils are fragrant, volatile compounds derived from a variety of plants, including flowers, herbs, spices, and trees. Aromatherapy works by stimulating the olfactory system, which is connected to the limbic system, the part of the brain that controls emotions. By inhaling the aroma of essential oils, the body is able to relax, reduce stress and promote healing.

Aromatherapy has many benefits, including improving mood, reducing stress, improving sleep, relieving pain, and boosting immunity. It can also help with relaxation and pain relief, and has been used to treat a variety of conditions such as headaches, skin problems, and digestive issues. Aromatherapy is safe and effective, and can be used in a variety of ways, such as through massage, baths, compresses, inhalations and diffusers. When using essential oils, it is important to be aware of their potential side effects, as they can irritate the skin and cause allergic reactions. People who are pregnant, have a medical condition, or are taking medication should consult a doctor before using aromatherapy. It is also important to use pure essential oils and to follow the directions carefully.

In conclusion, aromatherapy is a natural and safe form of healing that can be used to treat a variety of conditions. It is a great way to promote relaxation and reduce stress, and can be used in a variety of ways. However, it is important to be aware of potential side effects and to use pure essential oils. By following the directions carefully, aromatherapy can be an effective and safe way to promote healing and relaxation.